Your Health Matters

How to Achieve the Health
You Deserve in a Toxic World

Your Health Matters

How to Achieve the Health You Deserve in a Toxic World

By Dr. Tunis Hunt

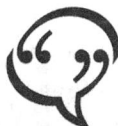

YouSpeakIt
PUBLISHING
The Easy Way
to Get Your Book
Done Right™

www.YouSpeakItPublishing.com

ISBN: 978-1-945446-20-7

Dedication

To all the amazing people who trusted me to join them on their health journey, for believing in themselves and that life is too short to not live at 100 percent.

For my life partner and greatest cheerleader — my wife, Estela, and the two people who inspire me to be my best — my children, Karis and Cooper.

Acknowledgments

You are the average of the five people you surround yourself with.

~ Jim Rohn

To my wife, Estela, for always allowing me to dream big and pursue my dreams, for allowing me the freedom to learn, travel, and grow into the man I am destined to be.

To my children, Karis and Cooper, who inspire me to be the best that I can be, for sharing me with the others whom I have had the privilege to serve.

To my parents for believing in me and for encouraging me to accomplish anything I put my mind to, for the provision and advantages that they have afforded me in life to become who I am.

To Carl, who helped me see who I am and the gift I had to share with the world, for opening my eyes to my potential and never allowing me to settle for less.

For the coaches, mentors, and colleagues who never gave up on me and constantly encouraged me to keep moving.

Contents

Introduction

I wrote this book to help you understand that your health is your greatest asset. I want to empower you with the tools, resources, and mindset to optimize your health. Too often, people are led to believe that their genetics or the circumstances of their environment control their health status. As a result, many rarely achieve the optimal level of health that they desire and deserve. This book was written as a guide to give those individuals who have the desire to live at their optimal health levels an opportunity to do so.

As a physician for over a decade, I have had the privilege of working with hundreds—if not thousands—of patients over the years. In that time, I have discovered that the most impactful element of an individual's quality of life is their health status. Poor health limits your ability, energy, and freedom to experience life as you desire.

How often has your ability to perform at your very best been impacted by your health?

How much better of a parent, spouse, employee, friend, and neighbor could you be if you weren't tired, depressed, anxious, achy, or battling the millions of other symptoms that plague our country?

Your health matters and when it is not at its best, you're not at your best. Many people have a desire to improve their health, yet are confused and uncertain about how to do so. The Internet, TV, radio, and print media produce an endless supply of information that is often misleading. Many people are running around in circles trying to figure out what to do and how to do it.

This abundant information can be conflicting and can cause you to become confused and indecisive, making it more difficult to achieve the health goals that you desire. This is the number-one complaint I hear from my patients who have tried to improve their health on their own. They are frustrated, confused, and overwhelmed about what to do and how to do it.

My goal is to dispel myths, reveal truths, and hopefully, open your eyes to a health approach that may be different from what you have heard up to this point. I ask that you read this book with an open mind and an open attitude. It is easy to fall prey to dogma, popular belief, what we see on TV, or what the so-called professionals tell us. Therefore, many of us continue to suffer because it may not be the best advice for us personally.

As you read, some of what I write here may:

- Challenge you
- Go against what you have been told in the past
- Make you question what you have been doing

That is all okay, because that is exactly the type of change in thinking and attitude that is required to get a different outcome than what you are currently getting.

My ultimate goal for you, the reader, is that you experience a paradigm shift regarding your health. I want you to understand the importance that it bears in your life, and support you in feeling you are empowered to control it. You don't have to be a victim of your health, but rather the designer of it. By implementing some of the mindset, suggestions, and tools in this book, I hope you will find that gaining and attaining the health goals that you want is not only possible, but it is something that you will enjoy achieving.

In Chapter One I discuss the epidemic we in this country currently face. We live in a world where disease is increasing despite the trillions of dollars spent annually on healthcare. The obvious question is: *why?* Chapter One shines a light on some of the biggest factors that are destroying our world and our health.

In Chapter Two we discuss our healthcare system. Does it really provide health?

What are some of the biggest misconceptions about health insurance, the FDA, and our healthcare providers?

We will dive into what must be done if you truly desire optimal health.

Chapter Three will provide you with a paradigm shift. It will explain why there is hope for you despite your current health status, medication use, or genetics. You will achieve the mindset necessary to achieve your health goals.

Once you have a new outlook, you need a plan. Chapter Four is that road map necessary to guide you. We will discuss what wellness looks like and why without it, you will never be able to achieve your health goals.

Chapter Five will give you a plan of action. Knowledge is worthless unless it can be applied, so this chapter provides action steps to get you moving toward the health goals you need.

I have been blessed to witness lives transform as individuals were able to understand information, follow a simple plan, and receive the support necessary for success. It is this experience that has birthed the passion in me to share this hope with the world. Everyone who has the desire can improve their health. This book is my effort to share this information with the masses.

CHAPTER ONE

The Epidemic

I will never forget receiving a dreaded phone call from my father. He shared with me that my mother had heard from her doctor and the tissue that they had routinely sampled from her breast proved to be cancerous. They were away on vacation and were having to cut their trip short to rush home and meet with the oncologist. He wasn't sure at the time, but felt that this was a serious life-threatening situation.

My parents returned and met with the doctor who explained that my mother would need to undergo both chemotherapy and radiation in hopes of saving her life. For the following months I had a front row seat to my mother's battle. My wife and I were between homes and as we were waiting on our new home to be built, we were living with my parents. So I saw firsthand my mother's body deteriorate due to the poisonous chemotherapy. I watched as she lost her energy, hair, and ability to enjoy life. As I witnessed this amazing strong woman succumb to this terrible disease, a passion was birthed inside of me. I wanted to help her out in any way that I could. I believed that there was information that could help her not only defeat cancer, but more important help her regain her health. So, I began my quest to discover the truth about disease, how our bodies work, and what can be done to maximize our health.

THE U.S. HEALTH EPIDEMIC

As I explored the data and the literature, I was shocked at what I discovered. I felt as if I had taken the red pill in the film *The Matrix*, and my perspective of the health of our nation, the role of government, big pharma, and the healthcare system completely changed. I quickly realized that much of the dogma that I had held as true was far from it. I learned that my mother's condition was far from rare and that one out of every eight U.S. women are diagnosed with breast cancer — approximately 300,000 new cases — every year![1]

Studying further, I discovered that despite the billions of dollars we spend on health-related expenses every year, in most major categories of chronic disease we were losing ground. Diabetes plagues 29 million people in the United States alone, and 70 million are believed to be pre-diabetic. Compare this to 1980 when there were only one million diabetics. Obesity now affects over half our population, including an alarming

---

1   breastcancer.org

number of children. Heart disease kills one out of every four people despite the trillion-dollar pharmaceutical industry fighting it. One out of every eight women will be affected with some sort of thyroid disease, adding to the epidemic of hormonal imbalances that the majority of U.S. women face.[2]

As I continued to read, I realized we have a health epidemic in our country, including high numbers of people who have:

- Autism
- Depression
- Anxiety
- Parkinson's
- Alzheimer's

There are also countless other diseases that our country faces.

ENVIRONMENTAL TOXINS

As I pondered the reality of this epidemic I asked myself: *How? Why?*

I quickly discovered that many things were probably responsible for our epidemic but none more so than the very things that we do to the food, water, and air that we so desperately need.

---

2 cdc.gov; niddk.nih.gov; thyroid.org

Environmental toxins are often a hidden factor in health status.

Toxins can be found everywhere:

- Sprayed on crops
- Released into the air
- Flushed into the water
- Slathered onto your skin as personal care products
- Wiped all over your home as cleaning products

These toxins and chemicals disrupt your body's natural ability to work.

Once you develop symptoms or concerns for your health, you may seek a diagnosis and medications. It is common to overlook environmental toxins, but you must implement awareness and strategies for dealing with these toxins to gain optimal health.

Herbicides and Pesticides

It's estimated that about a billion pounds of pesticides are used in the United States every single year, including:[3]

- Fifty-four different pesticides are found on spinach.

---

3   ephtracking.cdc.gov

- Twenty-six different pesticides are found on peaches.
- Research studies have shown forty-seven different residues on apples.[4]

Used to kill harmful bacteria and bugs that affect the plants, these poisons are massively ingested by the human population. As we eat crops laden with these chemicals, all types of problems can arise, including death. The World Health Organization estimates that there are three million cases of pesticide poisoning in the United States every year, accounting for over two hundred fifty thousand deaths.[5]

Other documented problems include:

- Memory loss
- Organization problems
- Motor skill problems
- Behavioral problems
- Asthma
- Allergies
- Hormone disruption
- Obesity
- Cancer

---

4 whatsonmyfood.org
5 who.int/mental_health/prevention/suicide/en/PesticidesHealth2.pdf

In addition, pesticides decrease the quality of our food. Industrialized farming and pesticide utilization deplete the nutrients in the soil resulting in produce with about half the nutrients of similar produce grown fifty or sixty years ago.6 It is the combination of ingesting these pesticides and the depletion of the nutrients that is wreaking so much havoc on our health and well-being.

On the other hand, produce grown with organic methods have very limited pesticide contact and that drastically reduces chemical exposure. Sustainable farming practices conserve the nutrients found in the soil, producing a more nutrient-dense product. This factor explains the importance of consuming organic produce or washing fruits and vegetables and buying meat and poultry raised in a sustainable manner. We may not be able to eliminate all the pesticides, but if we put a strategy in place to eliminate them to the best of our ability, it will go a long way in improving our health.

The Water Supply

Water is essential for life. As a human, you need to be consuming it the majority of your time. Unfortunately, water supplies, particularly in municipal areas, can be contaminated. Toxins such as fluoride, chlorine,

6 scientificamerican.com

radioactive contaminants, pharmaceutical drugs, lead, arsenic, and other pollutants are found in alarming quantities in our public water supplies.7 As a population, we are led to believe that these substances are there for public health and are in levels so low that they are not problematic to the body. Nothing could be further from the truth.

For example, the fluoride that is put into our water supply with the promise of healthy teeth is actually a waste product from the aluminum industry. Research clearly shows that it does not create healthy teeth but actually causes neurological damage.8 Chlorine is added to kill bacteria, but chlorine is not healthy to ingest. When you urinate after ingesting pharmaceutical drugs or wash pharmaceutical drugs down your toilet, it enters the water cycle and you ingest these drugs at alarming levels over time. Your skin is your biggest organ, allowing large quantities of these toxins to be absorbed when you shower and bathe.

A recent study found two hundred thirty-two foreign chemicals on average in the bodies of ten newborn babies.9 This proves just how prominent these chemicals are in our environment and how direct exposure is not even necessary to accumulate these poisons in our bodies.

---

7 ewg.org
8 fluoridealert.org
9 ewg.org

Reverse osmosis filtration systems installed at your sink or throughout your house remove the fluoride, chlorine, and pharmaceutical drugs. Strategies like this are excellent at reducing the toxins that you are exposed to every day. Many people use bottled water. I discourage this approach. Most bottled water is simply tap water. In addition, most bottled water is in plastic bottles which sit in hot warehouses, where additional toxins like BPA leach into the water. Buying a filtration system, whether as a point-of-service for your sink or showerhead, or ideally for a whole house, is the best strategy to lower the exposure to toxins. Carry water with you by investing in a glass or a stainless-steel container so you won't leach the toxins from a plastic container.

Personal Care Products

We often believe that if it's dangerous to drink that it's still okay to put on our body. We fail to realize that that is exactly what we do; we absorb that stuff through our skin. People don't realize just how many chemicals are used annually in personal care products. It is estimated that eighty-five thousand different chemicals are routinely used. What is more staggering is that less than three thousand of those eighty-five thousand are actually tested for safety measures. The worst part about it is none of them are tested synergistically, meaning Chemical A combined with Chemical B is never tested.[10]

If you turn over your shampoo bottle, you will notice it has more than one ingredient. It has ten, twelve, perhaps fifteen different ingredients. The Food and Drug Administration (FDA) does not regulate cosmetics and personal care products, except for colorizers in hair dye.[11] People don't realize that there is no government oversight for these products. It is up to the manufacturer to ensure they are safe to use.

Words like *natural* have little or no relevance on what the product actually contains. Still within those products you can find ingredients such as parabens, folates, petroleum, and fragrances. Many of these substances are known hormone disruptors. Estrogen-dominant cancers plague our society because of them. We are slathering them on our skin and hair and lips and eyelids.

A study led by the Environmental Watch Group in 2004 of more than two thousand participants estimates that, "The average woman uses 12 products containing 168 unique ingredients every day. Men, on the other hand, use 6 products daily with 85 unique ingredients, on average."[12] Many of the ingredients pose health

---

10 nrdc.org
11 fda.gov
12 ewg.org/skindeep/2004/06/15/exposures-add-up-survey-results/

risks to consumers, including cancers, and jeopardize the health of developing fetuses. If you are not aware of these ingredients, you can put a real burden on your detoxification pathways. To combat that, you need to use organic, natural products. The website, ewg.org/skindeep/, ranks your healthcare products and shows you how healthy the products you use are. It will help you determine alternatives that will be a better fit for your body.

CHRONIC STRESS

Many of us live in a fast-paced, never-resting environment. You may be constantly on the go, resulting in stress that depletes your body's ability to function at the optimal level.

In response to stress, the adrenal glands which sit atop your kidneys release several hormones, including:

- Epinephrine (adrenaline)
- Norepinephrine (noradrenaline)
- Cortisol

These hormones elicit a variety of physiological responses including the well-known fight-or-flight response. This response prepares your body for action, to either fight off the problem or to flee from it. This is a protective mechanism. The problem that lies in today's society is that this response is chronically *on*.

You may be moving from one stress to another in a typical day:

- Wake yourself up with an alarm
- Rush through breakfast
- Put makeup on in your car as you sit in traffic
- Use caffeine all day long

You may perpetually be under tremendous financial and emotional stress. As a result, your adrenal glands are forced to work overtime. This chronic response creates a perpetual inflammatory response in the body, creating an epidemic of stress-related health problems that are largely ignored by mainstream practitioners.

Emotional

There are three main sources of stress. The first one is *emotional stress*. Emotional stress is relational stress.

This is stress surrounding your relationships:

- Financial concerns
- Job struggles
- Studying
- Preparation for big events

Major relational experiences can take a toll on you.

Examples of these are:

- Loss of a loved one
- Divorce
- A new baby
- Moving

How they build upon each other is often overlooked. Research has shown that an emotional event you have lived through as far back as ten, fifteen, or even twenty years ago could still be impacting your health today.[13] If the health of your adrenal glands was not properly addressed and allowed to heal, these glands could still be working in a less than optimal capacity. This persistent stress will continue to be an underlying cause of inflammation in your body, causing multiple health concerns.

Toxins and Inflammation

As we discussed, toxins are everywhere in our environment. You must employ strategies to limit or avoid these toxins and regain your health.

Physical stress, such as aches and pain in your body, is also a major driver of stress and can be caused by:

---

13 ncbi.nlm.nih.gov/books/NBK207191/

- Poor posture
- Over-exercise
- Falls and accidents
- Lazy ergonomics

These culprits create a strain on your body that results in the inflammation mentioned previously. For many people, this is an everyday occurrence. This chronic activation of the adrenal system is a major burden that diminishes the quality of your health.

Health concerns include:

- Gastrointestinal disturbances
- Cardiovascular problems
- Memory loss
- Low libido
- Chronic fatigue

To regain your health, it is imperative that you address both physical stress and toxins.

You cannot eliminate every toxin in your environment, but taking the following steps are strides in the right direction:

- Eat organic foods.
- Use pure water.
- Use natural, organic personal care products.
- Practice proper posture and ergonomics.
- Exercise wisely.
- Get plenty of rest.

Dietary

Nothing impacts your health more than your food choices. The association between food and health is often overlooked or ignored. Most people struggle with the notion that the very things that they are putting into their mouths are the culprits to their health struggles. Instead, they look for every other excuse and rarely evaluate their diet.

The truth, however, is the food that you eat is what fuels your body with vitamins, nutrients, and minerals that your cells desperately need. When you eat foods dense in those nutrients, your cells receive lots of it. When you eat foods void of these — such as prepared or packaged foods — your cells are starved for nutrients.

When you eat products laden with sugar, artificial colors and flavors, and other chemicals, this is what your cells must use. Then, your cells do not operate at a high level. In addition, these chemicals are processed by your body, eliciting an adrenal response and inflammatory reaction. This inflammation is why many people may not have good energy, why so many struggle with sleep, and why millions struggle with concentration. Instead of looking for a pill or potion to fix these problems, simply evaluate the type of food you are putting in your system. This evaluation can offer tremendous results.

Of the major causes of stress on your body, your diet is the one you have 100 percent control over. Although you can put strategies in place to address the emotional, toxic, and physical stress, there will be limitations to what you can control. Your diet, however, is up to you.

CHAPTER TWO

The Healthcare Crisis

THE HEALTHCARE INDUSTRY DOESN'T PAY FOR HEALTH

In our country we not only have a health crisis; more specifically, we have a healthcare crisis. As I previously mentioned, in every major category of disease, we are going in the wrong direction. About one hundred seventeen million different people suffer from some type of chronic disease. Chronic disease can be defined as that type of disease which can and should be prevented and eliminated, yet seven out of every ten deaths in the United States are caused by these chronic diseases. Not only deaths, but as we get sicker, our quality of life deteriorates. It is estimated that every thirty seconds, a lower limb is amputated because of diabetic complications.[14] These are staggering statistics.

The United States spends about three trillion dollars in healthcare every single year—about ninety-five hundred dollars per person. Yet we are ranked number

14 cdc.gov/chronicdisease/overview/

thirty-seven in health by the World Health Organization despite spending a staggering two-and-a-half times more than any other country in the world.[15] The system is broken, and if we don't do something about it, then more and more people will get sicker.

Acute Care, Not Wellness

The United States has some of the brightest and best doctors in the world. Our schools do an amazing job at educating and equipping them to save lives. We have the best facilities, research departments, and medicines to deal with acute trauma care and disease management. Unfortunately, when it comes to wellness and prevention, our conventional healthcare system simply misses the mark. We train our doctors to function in this acute care model, yet we expect them to produce results that the system isn't designed to provide. It's not the doctor's fault. Our doctors are brilliant and well-meaning, but the system in which they are forced to work doesn't allow them to practice medicine the way most would like to. It's the system that is broken.

The system is designed for profit and efficiency. Visits are quick, symptoms are treated, and complaints dealt with as easily as possible, usually with a pill.

---

15   who.int/whr/2000/media_centre/press_release/en/; cms. gov/research-statistics-data-and-systems/statistics-trends-and-reports/nationalhealthexpenddata/downloads/highlights.pdf

Imagine for moment that your house was on fire.

Who would you pick up the phone and call?

The fire department, of course. And they would rush over with their axes and hoses and do their best to quickly put out the fire. Now, are they worried about wetting your carpet or breaking a window or door? Absolutely not — they are simply trying to put out the fire and they are the best in the world at doing so.

The next morning, the fire is out and the smoke has cleared. Are you going to call the same firefighters to come rebuild your house? Probably not.

You would call a contractor or handyman, someone with a completely different set of tools to achieve a completely different outcome. Yet, in our medical model, we are not doing this — we are not calling on the appropriate experts to help us maintain the best health. We are forcing our doctors to operate in a system designed for acute trauma care while expecting them to provide wellness and prevention, and it simply isn't working.

Is It Really Health Insurance?

When do you use your health insurance benefits?

Do you use them when you are healthy or sick?

Most insured people primarily use them when they are sick. You go to a doctor or have a procedure because of already-established symptoms or disease. Health insurance simply doesn't pay for prevention or wellness.

Health insurance provides as much health as life insurance provides life. It simply isn't designed to provide that to you.

I know you may be thinking: *What about mammograms, physicals, pap smears, and MRIs? Doesn't insurance pay for those procedures and aren't they prevention?*

Not really.

Think about this: Do these procedures prevent disease or do they simply detect what you already have?

Yes, they can be helpful in diagnosing a disease, but they do nothing toward *preventing* one. It is estimated that 90 percent of diseases today are not treatable with traditional, orthodox medical procedures. In other words, the very care you get from the procedures, pills, and potions that are offered in conventional medicine and paid for by your health insurance is not equipped to provide you health and wellness. Unfortunately, if you rely on your health insurance benefits for your health then you will simply never achieve it.

Symptom Relief Versus Fixing the Problem

Health insurance pays for drugs, surgeries, and quick doctor visits—thirteen to sixteen minutes being the most common length of visit reported in the United States in 2016.[16] None of these components provides you true health. It is a system designed to manage your concerns, not one designed to cure or prevent disease. Rarely does this system promote taking a step back to ask why the problem is occurring in the first place. Instead, it stops at suppressing or managing symptoms.

You have high cholesterol? There's a statin to lower it.

Hormones aren't balanced? Rub a cream into your skin.

Can't lose weight? Get a gastric bypass procedure.

Depressed? Take this medication to help with your happiness.

You could be on these medications every day for the rest of your life because if you quit taking these drugs, your symptoms would return.

In other words, the underlying root cause of the problem is never being addressed. Unfortunately, what so many people do in the United States is equate a pill to a skill. As long as their labs look good, or as

---

16 medscape.com (Medscape Physician Compensation Report, 2016)

long as the symptoms are suppressed, they believe they are healthy, not realizing that any problem that is left unaddressed only gets worse. This is why so many start out with one medication only to be placed on two, three, or four, and why you may have started with one symptom but now you have a whole list of symptoms. The underlying root cause is not being addressed.

The *Check Engine* Light

Medications in our culture are used like the check engine light in a car. Imagine you're driving your vehicle, and the check engine light comes on. Chances are you would take it to a mechanic to have your car evaluated and fixed.

Imagine if the mechanic simply popped open the hood, plugged his computer in and reset the light, turning it off and then sent you on your way.

What would most likely happen after driving around for a few miles?

The light would come back on.

Would you be willing to wake up every morning, drive your car to that mechanic, and have him turn off the check engine light?

I'm willing to bet you wouldn't. You probably would leave that mechanic, complaining about their inability to fix the problem, and find a new mechanic. The unfortunate truth is that every morning, millions of Americans wake up and turn off their check engine lights by taking their medications. And as a result, the root cause is never being addressed, thus more symptoms and more problems continue to manifest.

You must ask the better questions of why:

Why is my blood pressure high?

Why is my cholesterol level high?

Why is my thyroid not working?

Why is my gastrointestinal system not working?

Not until you address those root causes can you ever expect to achieve optimal health.

YOUR DOCTOR CAN'T FIX YOU

In the United States, we are blessed to have some of the best and brightest doctors in the world. Doctors choose their profession because they genuinely want to help people. In fact, most are forced to take very large loans to go through medical school, study countless hours, and dedicate a decade of their lives to achieve this goal. Unfortunately, despite their sacrifice, they find themselves trapped in what I consider a broken system, a system that is not solely dictated by the Hippocratic oath of *Do no harm*, but one that is persuaded by profit and big business.

Thus, many doctors struggle to provide the level of care that they desire to give. This system limits their time with patients, persuades their recommendations for care, and punishes them when their actions aren't aligned with those in charge. Therefore, despite our doctor's good intentions, you must learn to be your own health advocate.

A Broken System

The U.S. healthcare system is designed for profits. Publicly traded companies comprise our healthcare system. As a rule of thumb, their number-one obligation is to return a profit to the shareholders. Doctors are rewarded for doing procedures, prescribing medications, and for seeing as many patients as possible in a given time frame. Thus, the quality of care often goes down.

For instance, a doctor can spend fifteen minutes with you and put a stent in your heart and be paid up to ten thousand dollars. However, if they were to sit down with you for forty-five minutes and give you wellness goals and help you with a plan of action to achieve the same goal as the stent, they may get reimbursed fifteen dollars. The system simply isn't designed for wellness.

A Pill Doesn't Necessarily Equal Skill

There have been great advancements in medicine, and certainly medicine has proven to be life-saving in many instances. Most medication that is prescribed by doctors, however, is designed to manipulate symptoms and lab values, not actually address the root cause. Hence, in almost every situation, patients find themselves on these medications for the rest of their lives. Unfortunately, most doctors rely on medication as their main mode of treatment when it comes to your health.

Suppressing your symptoms or manipulating your lab values with medication is accepted as proper treatment by both the medical establishment and patients. However, many individuals fail to realize how much the manufacturers of these medications influence your doctor's decisions. Doctors are constantly visited by pharmaceutical sales reps who try to persuade them to use these products. Doctors are extremely busy and seldom have the time to do the necessary research on the products in the market and rely on these reps for information.

It is likely that as your doctor becomes more familiar with these reps and begins to trust them, they will be more prone to use a particular product. Pharmaceutical companies understand this brilliantly, and it is why they spend millions on employing reps. Unfortunately, many patients blindly accept whatever their doctor tells them and rarely question their doctor's approach and recommendations.

Just because the doctor can prescribe a medication that can manipulate the symptoms or lab values does not mean it is necessarily the most complete or the right thing to be done for your health. You may continue to suffer if that is all you accept.

You Are Your Best Doctor

No one cares more about your health than you do. It is vital that you take complete ownership of it. Often, we blindly give our ownership away, including to doctors, relinquishing the control of our health to what we believe to be their expertise and knowledge.

No one is going to be a better advocate for your health than you. You should be the one who takes responsibility for it by asking the right questions. A good healthcare practitioner encourages you to be an advocate for your health by inviting questions and conversation about their recommendations.

That is not always the case. Some practitioners become upset when a patient questions their judgment or asks about alternatives. The truth is you know your body better than anybody. You know what feels right and what does not feel right. Ask questions. Be the advocate for your health.

What Is Health Insurance, Really?

Health insurance was never designed to provide health to the masses. Health insurance was a concept originally offered by employers as a way for them to attract employees when there was a wage freeze during World Wars I and II.[17] Health insurance served as a way of increasing someone's compensation when raising salaries was forbidden.

As health insurance became more popular, it was primarily used to protect individuals from large medical expenses that could have led to financial hardships. It provided insurance from medical disasters. It was never created to pay for or limit our everyday medical care. Yet today much of our population relies on their health insurance policies to dictate their health decisions and people are rarely willing to invest in their own health. As a result, many struggle with achieving their health goals because insurance does not pay for wellness, but rather, it pays for disease management.

---

17 wikipedia.org (Health Insurance)

Your Insurance Company Is a Publicly Traded Company

Like the pharmaceutical companies, your health insurance provider is a publicly traded company that is obligated by law to make a profit for its shareholders. As a result, the policies, politics, and approved medical procedures are created with that in mind.

Health insurance companies maximize their profits by collecting higher premiums while restricting the benefits that they provide, such as:

- Limiting doctor reimbursements
- Denying procedures and labs
- Covering only certain medications

Despite paying thousands of dollars towards your health insurance every year, the quality of care that you receive is rarely the best:

- Your doctors can't spend the necessary time with you because they must see more patients.

- The most comprehensive labs aren't ordered because of managed care rules and regulations.

- Medications are prescribed for everything because it is the simplest and most time efficient approach to manage your concerns.

Your health suffers because of the restrictions your health insurance provider places on the healthcare system. Understanding this reality is crucial. If you allow your health insurance policy to dictate your healthcare decisions, then you will never reach your highest health potential.

You Don't Have to Let Them Dictate What You Can and Cannot Do

It is well established that insurance companies are restrictive in the benefits they provide, such as incomplete lab testing, generic medication, and rushed doctor's visits. You must be willing to take ownership of your health and seek opportunities to invest in it. Unfortunately, many individuals are not willing to do this. Because they have a health insurance policy that is supposed to pay for their health, they struggle with spending anything above and beyond. Thus, they continue to receive the same level of care that they have always experienced and, therefore, continue to struggle with their health.

No matter how much I believe that health insurance should pay for your health, it doesn't. It can provide some benefits, but your policy has limitations and if you want a different outcome from what it is providing, you must seek alternative approaches.

You Can Invest in Yourself

Your health is your most valuable asset.

When you have poor health, your quality of life suffers. You have the choice to view your health as an expense or an investment.

Either way, your health will cost you money. Too many Americans view health costs as an expense. They spend thousands of dollars every year on health insurance premiums, doctor visits, prescription medications, and procedures in reaction to health concerns as they arise. Fewer individuals strategically take a proactive approach to their health. As a result, millions of Americans find themselves running to providers, trying to manage their health concerns and symptoms.

This strategy not only costs the American people billions of dollars every year, but also has resulted in the rise of every chronic disease. It is estimated that the number one cause of bankruptcy among senior citizens in the United States is health-related problems.[18] It is also true that most of these people have health insurance.

Despite paying for and using their health insurance policies, insured people find themselves with prolonged health concerns and medical costs that they can't afford. Investing in your health and taking a proactive

---

18 debt.org/bankruptcy/statistics/

approach will save you money and allow you to enjoy the health that you desire.

So, what are some of the strategies you can start today to improve upon and prevent your health problems?

- Spend more money on your grocery bill by purchasing higher quality food.

- Join a gym.

- Buy supplements and vitamins recommended by a nutritionist or another qualified professional.

- Hire a coach, mentor, or healthcare provider who can give you guidance on preventative care.

Yes, it will require an investment. Yes, it will cost you time and money. But I promise it will be less than what you would spend if you get sick.

According to the American Diabetes Association:[19]

- Diabetics spend an average of $13,700 per year managing their disease.

- Chemotherapy treatment can cost up to thirty thousand dollars for eight weeks and then ten thousand dollars per week for oral medications.

---

19 diabetes.org

- A heart attack costs an average of $760,000 and ongoing medications can run someone with insurance $220.23 per month for the rest of their lives.

As you can see, spending a little more on proactive approaches will cost you far less than paying for sickness.

Health insurance should be reserved for catastrophes and not used as a guide of how to approach your health. It was designed to prevent you from going bankrupt if something serious happened and never designed to provide you health.

THE GOVERNMENT IS NOT RESPONSIBLE FOR YOUR HEALTH

The United States is the one of the greatest countries in the world. We have unbelievable opportunities and freedoms, as well as a government that cares for its citizens. Unfortunately, as great as our government is, it has many shortcomings.

Most people have the misconception that substances for sale, approved for medical treatment, and made available to the public have gone through tremendous testing and scrutiny, and that rigorous steps have been taken to ensure the substances or procedures are in fact the very best medicines for us citizens. Our government unfortunately does not have the resources or even the regulatory boards in place to do that effectively. In addition, lobbyists representing large corporations manipulate and pressure government agencies into allowing products and procedures to be available for the mere purpose of profit despite the potential harm or benefit they may have on the people.

The FDA

The origins of the Food and Drug Administration (FDA) can be traced back to 1906 when Theodore Roosevelt signed into law the Food and Drug Act also known as the Wiley Act—named after Harvey Wiley, its chief advocate. According to their website, www.fda.gov/AboutFDA/WhatWeDo/default.htm, the FDA is "responsible for protecting the public health by ensuring the safety, efficacy, and security of human and veterinary drugs, biological products and medical devices; and by ensuring the safety of our nation's food supply, cosmetics, and products that emit radiation."[20] The FDA is the watchdog that protects us from possible harmful products.

Despite good intentions, the FDA struggles to effectively scrutinize all the products that are introduced to the marketplace. In almost all instances,

---

20 fda.gov/AboutFDA/WhatWeDo/default.htm

the testing done on new products is not performed by independent government agencies but by the product manufacturers themselves. This practice provides an opportunity to manipulate data in favor of approval while diminishing the risks associated with it. As a result, medications, products, and chemicals that cause harm to our population are approved for use.

According to ProCon.org, a nonprofit nonpartisan public charity, the FDA has had to pull over thirty-five FDA-approved drugs off the market because they were proven to do more harm than good. Examples include Baycol and Vioxx, which have been linked to over two hundred forty thousand deaths combined in the four short years they were on the market.

According to a 2014 investigative study by Genevieve Pham-Kanter, of the decisions made by the FDA between the years of 1997–2011, more than 13 percent of the time the voting committee members had financial interests in the drug that was being approved.[21] In addition, there have been numerous high-ranking FDA employees who were either once employed by large chemical or pharmaceutical companies or who left the FDA to go work for these companies. It is estimated that during the last decade alone, over seven high-ranking FDA officials have worked for Monsanto. Talk about a conflict of interest!

---

21 milbank.org/quarterly/articles/revisiting-financial-conflicts-of-interest-in-fda-advisory-committees/

The Lobbyists

Over the last decade, it is estimated that at any given time there are over ten thousand lobbyists in Washington, DC, working to influence the decision makers. In 2010, lobbyists spent over $3.52 billion attempting to persuade our legislators to allow, prevent, or keep special interests that would help their clients improve their profits.

Lobbyists also play a large role when it comes to influencing the decisions the FDA makes concerning what is approved for market. Over the past decade, an average 397 full-time lobbyists have been dedicated to influencing the decisions of the FDA every year. Thus, many products, chemicals, and medications are approved for use that provide more profit than they do benefit to the American people.[22]

A good example is the tobacco industry. For decades, the public was kept in the dark about the harmful effects of cigarette smoking due to lobbyists influencing our policy makers. And although it has been well established that cigarette smoking is harmful to your health, in 1998 the tobacco industry spent over thirty million dollars lobbying decision makers about their products. Simply put: *money talks.*

---

22 opensecrets.org

Your Best Advocate Is You

As convenient as it would be to allow the government to assume the role of your health advocate, it simply isn't a wise choice if optimal health is your desire. Because of companies motivated by profit and government officials motivated by power, your best interests are rarely considered.

The only way to ensure that your health is optimized is to be willing to take responsibility for it. This includes scrutinizing the products recommended, medications prescribed, and the dogma presented by conventional medicine, media, and industry. The good news is with the Internet, books, podcasts, and videos, there is no better time in history to discover information. If you are willing to educate yourself, question what is being presented, and ask better questions, achieving your health goals is only a matter of time.

CHAPTER THREE

You Can Achieve Health

YOUR BODY IS INTELLIGENTLY DESIGNED

Have you ever wondered why simply putting a bandage over a cut is often all that is required to heal it?

Why does your body produce a fever when there is an infection present?

Why do you get nauseated when you ingest something that is harmful to your health?

It is because you are an intelligent, self-healing organism. When your body is working at an optimal level, you enjoy abundant energy, vitality, and happiness.

Unfortunately for many, this is not the case. Millions are plagued with poor health and the struggles that it creates. They are led to believe that their genetics and circumstances have them trapped with their symptoms and diseases and there is no real hope for them to achieve better health. Despite their current health condition, the amount of medications they may be on, or how many other family members currently struggle with the exact same thing – there is hope.

You Can Thrive

Imagine for a moment that you came to my office and noticed a wilted plant sitting in my waiting room. Now imagine that I approached you and asked for your advice on how I can help my plant thrive again.

What suggestions would you give?

I am willing to bet that you would suggest things like water, sunlight, fertilizer and nutrients, and maybe even recommend that I evaluate the soil for bugs or toxins, or suggest that I re-pot it.

Now imagine I followed your advice, what will most likely happen to my wilted plant?

I believe that we would agree it would thrive again. In other words, if I gave the plant what it needed and took away some of the things it didn't need, the plant inherently knows how to thrive and be healthy again. This same principle holds true with the human body.

If you give the body what it needs — proper nutrients, water, sunlight — and take away some of the things it doesn't need — artificial colors and sweeteners, too much stress, alcohol, and sugar — your body will thrive again. Too often, however, we lose sight of this and forget how the choices that we make every day play an important role in the status of our health.

It's Not a Lack of Medicine

In our society, when people get a symptom or diagnosis, the first thing they typically consider is: *What do I have, and what can I take for it?*

In fact, WebMD.com is the number-one medically ranked website because of their symptom search function. We are programmed to think that our bodies have some sort of deficiency that must be addressed. Unfortunately, in most cases, we assume some sort of medication is what we need. For instance, if you get a headache, you may take ibuprofen or acetaminophen.

But have you ever evaluated that logic?

It is as if we are telling ourselves: *I am running low on ibuprofen in my body so adding some back will fix my problem.*

Instead, you could take a step back and ask why the headache was there in the first place:

- Too much stress?
- Lack of water?
- Lack of sunshine?

Whatever you are suffering with: constipation, high cholesterol, high blood pressure, and so forth, if your thought process is: *The body must be lacking something; therefore I need to put something that is man-made into it to make it work better,* then you will fail to discover the root cause of your concerns.

If you take the time to dive deeper, take a step back and ask the *Why* question:

- Why is my cholesterol high?
- Why do I have high blood pressure?
- Why do I have this headache?
- Why are my hormones not balanced?

If you incorporate this method of thinking you will find the root causes of your health concerns and the answers will help you achieve the health goals you desire.

You Are a Self-Healing, Vitalistic Organism

As I mentioned earlier, I believe the body is intelligently designed, and it is capable of self-healing and self-regulation. The term *innate* is often used to describe the body's ability to intelligently operate without assistance. For instance, we don't think about our breathing or our heart beating or a lot of the processes the body goes through because it is automatic. It is the autonomic nervous system running. It is smarter than we are.

The body is always trying to return to equilibrium or *homeostasis.* For instance, if there is a bacterial infection in your body wreaking havoc, your body creates a fever to destroy those bacteria. You may try to be smarter than the body and pop a pill to bring down a fever. By doing that, however, you're getting in the way of your body's own healing. When you reduce the fever, you reduce the body's ability to kill off the bacteria. Therefore, you invite an ongoing infection.

If I get a minor cut on my finger or my hand, I will initially put some pressure on it to bring the bleeding to a stop. But I don't have to do anything about healing. I don't have to tell the body how to regenerate tissue. I don't have to tell the body anything, and it returns to a state of perfection all on its own.

YOUR HEALTH HAS MORE TO DO WITH YOUR DECISIONS THAN YOUR GENETICS

Many of my patients come to me with the belief that they can only manage or make the best of living with a condition or set of systems. They think that because they have suffered for some years with it, or because they're on five, six, or ten different medications, or because everybody in their family currently suffers with it, that it's unreasonable to think they could feel better.

These patients don't have true hope of achieving their health goals. Sure, maybe they can have some improvements, but living at their optimal, ideal health is outside of their perceived reality.

Epigenetics Control Genes

Epigenetics is the study of biological mechanisms that switch genes on and off. Certain circumstances in life can cause genes to be silenced or expressed over time. In other words, they can be turned off—become dormant, or turn on—become active.

Epigenetics are everywhere:

- What you eat
- Where you live
- Who you interact with
- When you sleep
- How you exercise
- How you age

All these can eventually cause chemical modifications around the genes that will turn those genes on or off over time.

How your genes behave are also affected by outside factors:

- Toxin
- Diet
- Stress
- Trauma

There are countless reasons why these genes get turned on and off. The exciting reality of epigenetics is that you don't have to be a victim of your genetics. You have the power to influence your health.

You can support your genes in many ways:

- Eating a good diet and the right nutrients
- Getting proper rest and sleep
- Keeping your stress levels in check
- Controlling exposure to environmental toxins

These are some of the ways you can determine your health destiny. Epigenetics are reversible.

With twenty thousand-plus genes, what will be the result of the different combinations of genes being turned on or off?

The possible permutations are enormous! But if we could map every single cause and effect of the different combinations, and if we could reverse the gene's state to keep the good while eliminating the bad, then we could slow aging, stop obesity, and do so much more. This means that just because you have a certain gene, it is not automatic that you will manifest a trait.

Siblings and Twins

To drive home epigenetics, we can explore why siblings or identical twins often have different health statuses. It's not because their genes are different. It's not because they don't have the same chromosomes or gene makeup. It's how they have taken care of themselves or how they have experienced life that has manifested those genes turning on or off. In fact, it is a well-researched conclusion that identical twins rarely struggle or die of the same disease.[23]

The Power of Choices

It is well researched that your current health status has more to do with the choices that you've made than your genetics.[24] Whether you are happy, indifferent, or displeased with your current health status, it is a result of your choices. What's empowering, however, is knowing that if you are unhappy and want to change, you have the power to do so.

To experience a different health status requires better and most likely different choices than you are currently making.

Embrace a determined mindset and find:

- What foods serve your body?
- What types of exercise are best for your body?
- How can you incorporate rest, relaxation, and meditation?

23 theguardian.com/science/2013/jun/02/twins-identical-genes-different-health-study
24 www.sciencedaily.com/releases/2011/02/110207112539.htm

The choices you make every day will influence the quality of your health.

You may think: *I just got sick overnight,* or *I had a really bad month,* or *I don't know how my health status got to this point.*

But a shift in major illness rarely happens overnight. Disease more likely results from a combination of daily choices we make over the course of weeks, months, and years. Putting a game plan in place will make a huge difference in your health if it's not where you want it to be.

DESPITE HOW LONG YOU'VE SUFFERED, THERE'S HOPE

Expecting Different Results from the Same Actions Is Crazy

Despite how long someone has struggled with their current health condition, how many medications they may be on, or how many other family members currently suffer with the exact same thing, there is hope!

You can improve your health. You can reduce or eliminate medications and achieve health goals that you once thought impossible. Having said that, there is a catch: for you to achieve a different health status than you are currently experiencing, *you must be willing to do something different than you are currently doing.* Albert Einstein is credited with saying, "Doing the same thing over and over again expecting different results is insanity." There is absolutely no way that you will be able to achieve a different health status if you are unwilling to make a change in what you are doing.

Different Approach

We have already established that our current healthcare system is in real trouble:

- Despite the billions of dollars that are spent every year, *thousands out of your own pocket,* we are going in the wrong direction in every category of chronic disease.

- Health insurance doesn't actually pay for wellness or prevention, but rather acute trauma care.

- A practitioner has good intentions but is unable to provide the level of care which is often necessary.

- Medications and procedures simply mask the symptoms and ignore the root underlying causes.

If wellness is your desire, you must step outside of this broken system and be willing to invest your own time, energy, and finances to achieve it. In other words, you need to stop pretending that simply going to your primary care practitioner and using your health insurance benefits will get you the level of health you desire. A different approach is necessary. A doctor with a different set of skills is necessary. A completely different mindset is necessary.

It' Not Too Late

One of the greatest joys I experience as a physician is watching individuals achieve their health goals. I have been blessed to witness hundreds of lives change over the past decade and each one holds a special place in my heart. One experience is very special to me. I had the privilege to work with a wonderful woman named Elma. When I met Elma, she was seventy-nine years old. She had suffered from type 2 diabetes for forty years. She was on seven different medications, six of them for diabetes, one for cardiovascular health. In addition, almost 80 percent of her family suffered from type 2 diabetes.

Over the course of the last forty years, Elma had battled diabetes and despite taking the medications and following her doctor's advice, she was unsuccessful in lowering her fasting blood glucose levels below three hundred — normal fasting glucose is ninety-five or lower.

Instead of giving up, Elma had hope that her body could heal if the right approach was taken for her health. We ran some comprehensive labs to discover all her health concerns, and she allowed us to show her how to eat, how to exercise, how to take care of her body.

Within three weeks, she had to cut back half her medication. Her blood glucose levels, which had never been under three hundred, were down into the one-fifties! Six months later, she was down to one medication and now, she has almost completely normal blood glucose.

If Elma, at age seventy-nine, with type 2 diabetes, on seven different medications, and a family history of diabetes can improve her health, don't you agree that you can do it as well?

CHAPTER FOUR

The Wellness Approach

ALL SYSTEMS FUNCTION AS ONE

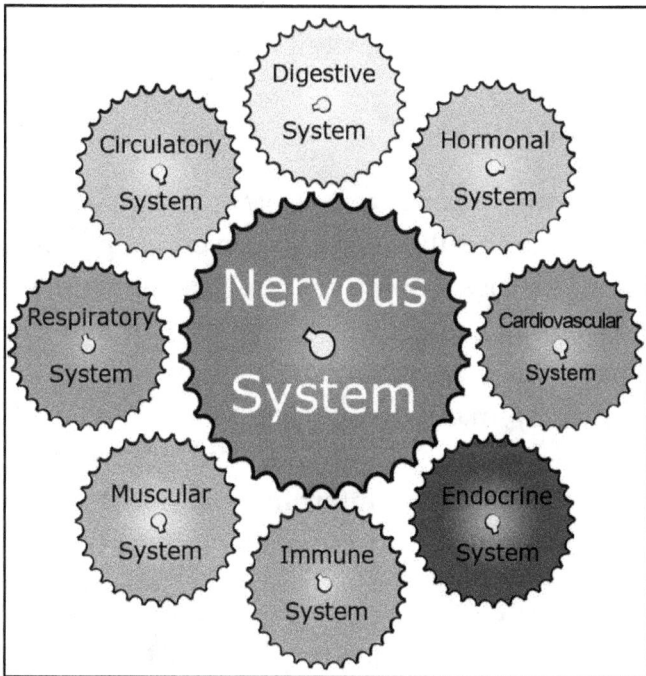

Conventional medical approaches do a poor job at improving most chronic health conditions that plague so many Americans. Illnesses are simply managed and rarely is a plan of action to reverse or eliminate the disease put into action. This is a tragedy! Not only is the quality of these individuals' lives diminished, but they are left with no hope to heal.

Our bodies were intelligently designed, and if given the opportunity, they will thrive. As introduced in the previous chapter, to thrive you must be willing to take a proactive approach to wellness that gets to the root cause so that you can maximize your health.

Like a Swiss Watch

You are a complex, comprehensive organism. Your body is comprised of trillions of cells, seventy-eight organs, and twelve major systems that all must work together. Each cell, organ, and system relies on communication with each other to create your existence. It is silly to think that by manipulating, influencing, or working on one area of your body you wouldn't be affecting another part as well. Unfortunately, this principle is often forgotten when addressing your health.

Healthcare providers who specialize in one aspect of health—cardiologists, gastroenterologists, endocrinologists—will treat you specifically for that system and give little thought for the other systems in the body. You find yourself running to one doctor for one type of treatment or medication and then running to another for another procedure or medication. Rarely are your doctors working together to come up with a comprehensive plan to improve your health. Thus, you find yourself on multiple medications, continuing to suffer with symptoms, and no real understanding on how to achieve your health goals.

THE FIVE GEARS OF HEALTH

A better approach would be one in which your health was comprehensively evaluated, one that looks at your systems as one whole and identifies all the underlying root concerns. Then a plan of action could be put into place that addressed all these concerns simultaneously.

There are five key components that must be addressed.

I refer to these components as the *Five Gears of Health*:

- Detoxification
- Nutrition
- Exercise
- Hormones
- Nervous System

Based on my decade of work with patients, it is only when all these gears are addressed is it possible to truly regain your health. Just like a well-crafted Swiss watch requires all its gears to turn in order to function, the same is true of making progress in your health. If just one area is not properly evaluated and improved upon, then the desired outcome is missed.

Detoxification

Nothing is as fundamental as detoxification or cleaning out the junk in your system. As we have already discussed, the environment is loaded with chemicals and other toxins that your body must deal with. In addition, you may eat foods, drink water, and take medications that are loaded with substances your body was never designed to ingest.

Pathways to detoxification include your:

- Liver
- Kidneys
- Gut
- Skin
- Breath

Over time, these organs can get bogged down and work less efficiently. The toxins and pollutants accumulate in your body and create symptoms. Only when you effectively eliminate these toxins from your body do you set yourself up for healing. Failure to do so results in perpetual struggles despite your other healthy changes.

For example, if you never changed the air filters in your home, would it matter if you updated your air system to improve its function? Probably not. As long as the filters were covered in dust, blocking the flow of air, changing the entire system would provide little improvement. Similarly, if you simply change your eating, exercise, or other health habits but haven't effectively cleaned out the junk, then you will most likely continue to struggle.

What do I mean by detoxification?

I am not suggesting a colon cleanse or going to the local store and buying a shake that makes you sit on the toilet for the next few days. I am suggesting that you work with a healthcare professional to properly elicit both Phase One and Phase Two detox pathways so that you reap the benefit that you are looking for.

> **Phase One:** this pathway converts a toxic chemical into a less harmful chemical. This conversion is achieved by various chemical reactions such as oxidation, reduction, and hydrolysis.

> **Phase Two:** this pathway is called the *conjugation pathway*, whereby the liver cells add another substance such as cysteine, glycine, or a Sulphur molecule to a toxic chemical or drug, to render it less harmful. This addition makes the toxin or

drug water-soluble, so it can then be excreted from the body via watery fluids such as bile or urine.

In our clinic, we typically prescribe for our patients a specific diet that is easy to follow and provides nutrients to support those pathways.

Nutrition

Food is fuel. Just like the plant needs certain vitamins, minerals, and nutrients to thrive; so does your body. You get these through your food choices. Make the right choices and your body thrives. Make poor decisions, and your body suffers. According to the Macmillan Dictionary, *food* is defined as "that which is eaten to sustain life, provide energy, and promote growth and repair of tissues."

Do you think fast food cheeseburgers fit that definition?

What about diet soda?

Of course not! We all inherently know that some foods are better than others, but often we do not choose wisely.

Why?

Would you fill up your vehicle which requires unleaded gasoline with diesel fuel?

What if I paid you $100 to do so?

You wouldn't even consider it. You understand what the wrong fuel does to your vehicle's engine and the cost required to fix it.

The same is true with your body. When you consistently put the wrong foods—like artificial sweeteners, food dyes, sugar, hydrogenated fats and oils—in your body, it too will be destroyed and require tremendous expense to fix it. One of the most fascinating aspects of working with individuals is to watch their health transform as they make simple dietary changes from those which were causing damage to those that provide the correct fuel their bodies need.

Food is powerful. It can be either powerfully good or powerfully bad. The choice is yours.

Hormones

Experts believe that there are over fifty different hormones in your body which are responsible for thousands of processes every second.[25] Hormones have been tied to thousands of symptoms and play a large role in your health concerns, whether related to sleep, energy, mental abilities, or losing weight.

---

25 ikonet.com

In order to get in the shape that you want and stay in that shape, you must have properly functioning hormones. There are fat-storing hormones: estrogen, cortisol, and insulin. There are also fat-burning hormones: growth hormone, thyroid, and testosterone. In addition, depending on what hormone is imbalanced, you will struggle with body fat.

Properly testing hormones is not commonly done. At best, your doctor may run a simple blood panel to look at estrogen, progesterone, or testosterone, but it is unlikely that they'd look at all the other important factors that influence these hormones.

Two hormonal glands that tend to be overlooked are the adrenals and the thyroid. Although some allopathic healthcare providers will test your thyroid, it is usually not a comprehensive test.

Thyroid metabolism is complex, and testing TSH—a pituitary hormone—alone is never enough to properly evaluate your thyroid function. When providers stop there, it leaves millions of men and women suffering with thyroid-related symptoms despite medication or having *normal* lab values.

The adrenal glands are rarely evaluated in conventional medicine. Unless there is suspicion of severe adrenal disease, most doctors simply ignore its role in your health. The adrenal gland, as you will remember, is responsible for responding to stress in your life. It is ludicrous to think that stress plays no role in your health. Only when your adrenal glands are properly evaluated and supported can you expect to have normal hormone function.

This is one of the biggest differences in my work with patients; I see positive results in an individual's health when their adrenals are taken care of.

Exercise

A good friend of mine once explained, "I don't exercise because weights are heavy and running makes me tired."

While this was meant to be humorous, it is how many people perceive exercise. The importance of exercise is something that most elementary school kids understand and one that all of us inherently know. We should dedicate more time to being active. *Lack of time* is one of the most prevalent excuses individuals use for why they don't regularly exercise. Next on the list is *lack of results* and *feeling worse when I do exercise*.

Exercise is extremely important in achieving health, but I understand why most people don't incorporate it in their lives. With thousands of workouts to choose from, it can be incredibly confusing to know the right one for you. Many find themselves perpetually spinning their wheels, only to be frustrated by the lack of results. The key to exercise is to work out smarter not harder.

Identify what will help your body burn fat, not just use up your energy. In some cases, this may require a higher intensity pace of workout, and in others, it will require a slower, restorative pace of workout. This is where testing your hormones and working with a trainer can be helpful in achieving your goals.

I have seen individuals who exercised with high intensity five days a week and struggled to get results finally achieve their goals when they completely switched to a slower approach. Others have added a session or two of resistance training and that was the difference they needed to break through that weight loss plateau.

The bottom line is that exercise is necessary, but only if it is smartly designed for you.

Nervous System

The nervous system is your master system. It comprises your brain, spinal cord, and nerves. It is how your body communicates. If there's a compromise in how this system is working, you experience health struggles and symptoms. The biggest culprit is inflammation. Inflammation has been linked to every chronic disease that is known, and when it is present, your body is under extreme stress trying to compensate for it.[26] Despite its large role in your health, inflammation is seldom emphasized by doctors as a key component to your health concerns. It is rarely looked for in lab testing and when suspected, simply suppressed with medications and steroid injections.

Only when inflammation is properly identified and addressed will you achieve optimum health.

Some of the biggest influences of inflammation are:

- Food
- Exercise
- Stress

Another step you can take in ensuring neural health is to make sure that any interference of your spinal information highway is removed. Chemical, emotional, and physical stress on your body can negatively affect the mobility and function of your vertebral column.

The vertebral column is the set of vertebra, or back bones, that protects your spinal cord and provides you with the ability to stand upright as well as bend and twist. When restriction occurs due to stress, inflammation can develop on the nerve roots exiting the foramen, or holes, between your vertebra and cause improper nerve signaling.

---

26 sciencedaily.com

Symptoms of impeded nerve signaling include:

- Muscle spasms
- Numbness
- Tingling
- Pain

As well, more serious or systemic problems can occur:

- Constipation
- Rapid heartbeat
- Asthma

Properly restoring the function of these joints is necessary for optimal health.

To ensure these joints function at their highest capacity, you can seek:

- Chiropractic adjustments
- Acupuncture
- Massage

I am often amazed at the healing changes achieved when individuals simply add routine chiropractic adjustments to their wellness plan.

Only when you spin all these gears can you expect to achieve optimal health. Many individuals have come to my office claiming to have worked on one of these areas in the past with limited or no results. When only one or two of these gears were addressed, ignoring the others, the patient continued to suffer with symptoms. If complete health is your desire, you must be willing to address all these gears.

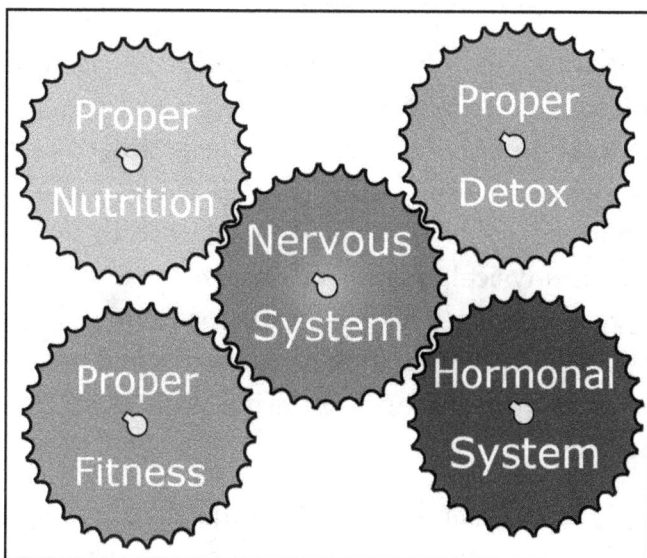

BETTER LAB TESTING

Lab testing is a tool used by doctors that helps identify problems you may be experiencing. Many practitioners neglect to use the latest and greatest labs available. Due to practice management policies and insurance restrictions, well-meaning physicians are limited in what diagnostic testing they can order. This can result in very basic—and in many instances, outdated—lab testing, leaving many individuals suffering with chronic problems.

The Problem With Conventional Lab Testing

Lab testing in conventional medicine is highly standardized. Policies, politics, and financial consideration play large roles in the standard of care that physicians are encouraged to follow. The bare minimum is typical for screening your health. For most people, a physical exam is all they receive when they visit their doctors. This basic panel is reviewed and if everything happens to look good, nothing else is done. This leaves many people suffering with unaddressed symptoms.

One of the largest concerns of standardized lab testing is the lack of specificity it provides. When you go to your doctor and they order a lab test, after samples are collected and analyzed, you get a report that shows your values. Next to your values is a *reference range* of numbers that your value is compared to. If your value falls within that range then you are considered healthy, but if it is currently outside of that range, your practitioner may show some concern.

Have you ever considered how lab companies come up with that reference range?

Reference ranges are created by averaging the lab values of the population, more specifically, the population of a particular region or state. For instance, in the state of North Carolina, the reference range used on lab testing is made up of the values of individuals tested in that state, which are then pooled and averaged. A Bell curve is used to place 95 percent of those values under it as normal leaving a 2.5 percent deviation on either end. In other words, this method assumes that 95 percent of the population is healthy.

Do you actually think 95 percent of the population is healthy?

Who typically gets tested, sick or healthy people?

This method also creates differences in ranges from state to state. For instance, you could get tested in North Carolina, jump on a plane to Texas, get the same labs and be given different results.

That doesn't seem very scientific, does it?

What about your value as it compares to the range?

Have you ever had a value at the very top or bottom of the normal range?

For example, if the reference range for normal was 25–55 md/dl and your value was 55, an allopathic doctor may not discuss this with you because it technically falls into the normal range, despite being only one point away from abnormal.

Functional Lab Testing: A Better Approach

Functional lab testing, on the other hand, can provide you with better answers and a proactive approach. We like to think of it as putting the yellow light into lab testing. Imagine if all intersections had traffic lights that went from green to red.

What would most likely happen in many of those intersections?

Crashes and chaos.

Having a yellow light allows a warning that the traffic pattern is about to change and provides drivers an opportunity to react accordingly. This is the same philosophy functional doctors use when evaluating lab values. Instead of simply relying on the reference ranges, functional doctors use healthy ranges. They look for patterns and concerns to offer guidance to patients *before* a major problem occurs. For example, if the reference range for TSH is .45 to 4.5 uU/ml, and your result was between those two points, then your doctor would most likely tell you there is no thyroid concern.

Functional doctors, however, understand that true thyroid health typically occurs when your TSH levels are between 1.8 and 3.0. So if your value is 3.5 or 1.5, for example, a functional doctor may take a proactive approach to start addressing your thyroid health instead of waiting until it moves beyond the reference ranges. They put the yellow light into lab testing to offer a warning and an opportunity to address concerns before they become problems.

TSH Value

| -------------------- | -------------------- | -------------------- |
.45   (yellow)   1.8 (Healthy Range) 3.0   (yellow)   4.5

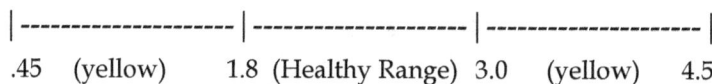

As valuable as blood testing can be, it is not without limitations. When evaluating hormones and gut health, for example, simple blood testing doesn't provide a complete picture of your health. Hormones can be either *bound*—connected to a transport molecule—or *unbound*—free, not connected. The most active form of a hormone is the unbound form. Blood testing does not allow evaluation of most unbound hormone forms. You are left with incomplete answers to your hormone health.

Another example of the limitations of blood testing is in evaluating how stress is affecting your health. Cortisol, the stress response hormone, naturally fluctuates throughout the day. It is typically highest in the morning and lowest prior to bedtime. To properly evaluate this fluctuation or *circadian rhythm*, you would need a method that would allow you to provide several samples throughout the day. Because collecting multiple blood samples through the day would inconveniently require a day-long clinic setting, hormonal levels are instead tested by collecting saliva or urine, which you can easily do on your own at home or work. This type of testing is not only more informative, but also allows a physician to be much more accurate in addressing your health concerns.

Answers Equal Results

Results occur only when the underlying cause is properly evaluated and addressed. Let's return to the example of thyroid testing. In the United States, the standard of care is to evaluate a number called TSH, thyroid stimulating hormone. This hormone is the only marker your doctor is required to evaluate to diagnose you with a thyroid disorder and place you on medication for the rest of your life.

Thyroid metabolism, however, is much more complicated than that. To start with, The TSH that your doctor evaluates is actually a pituitary hormone. Your doctor makes assumptions about your thyroid health based on a pituitary hormone! In truth, your thyroid actually produces hormones of its own. The most prominent two are T4 and T3.

Wouldn't it make more sense to evaluate those?

In addition, T4 and T3 aren't created equal. Think of T4 as *crude oil* and T3 as *gasoline*.

Which drives your car, *crude oil* or *gasoline*?

Gasoline does. The same is true for thyroid metabolism, T3 is the active form the body wants. And to make matters more complicated, most of the T3 your body uses isn't made by your thyroid but instead is a result of T4 being converted into T3 in areas like your liver and gut. *Good functioning liver and gut health (detoxification) are important for thyroid health.*

Just like other hormones, T3 can be bound or un-bound. It is the un-bound form that attaches to the DNA receptor sites of your cells. As you can see, your thyroid health is much more complicated than a simple TSH value. To accurately evaluate your thyroid health, you need to look at multiple markers including Total T4 and T3, Free T4 and T3, Reverse T3, and antibody markers like Thyroid Peroxidase (TPO) Ab and Antithyroglobulin Ab.

It is estimated that 60 percent to 90 percent of hypothyroidism cases in the United States are actually a result of an autoimmune disease known as Hashimoto's

Hypothyroidism. This means your thyroid isn't the true problem, but your immune system is. In the case of Hashimoto's, your immune system is attacking the thyroid tissue, causing thyroid disruption and symptoms. The medication often prescribed for thyroid health completely ignores this mechanism, leaving individuals struggling with thyroid symptoms despite normal labs.

A prime example of this is our work with our patient, Nora. She was diagnosed with hypothyroidism and, despite being on medication and having normal labs, she struggled with weight gain, fatigue, and low energy for over fifteen years. She was constantly going to her doctor and having her levels checked.

Repeatedly, her doctor told her that her thyroid was under control because her lab values were normal and that her symptoms must be a result of something else. Eventually, her doctor suggested that her symptoms were all in her head and prescribed antidepressant and anti-anxiety medication.

Thankfully for Nora, she didn't give up and eventually learned that there were options that she hadn't explored yet. After learning about our unique approach, she agreed to partner with us. We immediately ordered a complete thyroid panel that clearly showed that she had Hashimoto's. In addition, we evaluated her diet, adrenal health, and inflammatory markers. Within sixty days of addressing her root cause, she had lost thirty pounds, her cholesterol had normalized, she was able to cut her medication by half, and she was full of energy.

Lab testing can be your best friend or your most frustrating enemy. If you find yourself struggling with symptoms and your lab values are normal, then better testing must be ordered. Unfortunately, some of the most accurate and complete testing isn't covered by your health insurance policy. Many doctors may not even be comfortable ordering them.

You must become your own advocate by:

1) Finding physicians who are willing to think outside the box

2) Taking responsibility for investing in your own health

CHAPTER FIVE

Health Is Not an Accident; It's a Design

DECIDE TO BE HEALTHY

The quality of your health will directly influence the quality of your life. When you are in good health you are a better spouse, parent, friend, neighbor, and co-worker. When your health is compromised, you may find yourself struggling to be what you were created to be.

Good health does not just happen. You will need to decide that health is important and put the steps and processes in place to achieve it.

Sick and Tired of Being Sick and Tired

Many individuals claim they want to be healthy, but it is not until someone is sick and tired of being sick and tired that they implement the necessary steps to achieve their health goals. Although many Americans have arrived at this point and are searching for answers, there are plenty of people who are not quite at this point. They approach their health passively without intention or a plan. They place little thought on the foods they consume, their sleep habits, or their activity level throughout the day. They succumb to simply taking medication and living with their health status and symptoms. As a result, they never achieve the goals they want. The enemy of great is good, and many people walk around with good health instead of claiming what is inherently theirs — great health.

To Get a Different Result, You Must Do Something Different

Remember, if you truly are unhappy with your current health status and desire a different outcome, you are going to have to figure out what you need to do different.

Is it a different way of eating?

Is it seeing a different healthcare practitioner?

Or is it completely changing your mindset and approach to your health?

As stated before, research shows that your current health status relies on your choices, not your genetics. If you are willing to decide to be healthy, you absolutely can achieve it. Don't settle for your current status if it is not where you want it to be. Figure out what needs to be done, and be willing to put the steps in place to achieve it.

DEVELOPING A PLAN

> *Failure to plan is a plan to fail.*
> ~Benjamin Franklin

You must be willing to design and implement a plan if you truly desire change in your health. Desired results don't just happen, they are designed. Only when you prioritize your health goals and implement a plan of action to achieve them will you move in your desired direction.

No More Excuses, Just Go for It

It is tempting to limit our responsibility by blaming our genetics or circumstances.

There are many excuses you can use to rationalize why you aren't enjoying the quality of health you want:

- Family history
- A previous diagnosis
- Medication use
- Finances
- Time
- Where you live

The quality of your health is a direct result of the decisions that you make daily.

Now, I understand that you don't always feel like doing the right thing. Eating fast food is more convenient; staying up late to watch a show is enjoyable; it is easier to sleep in rather getting up early to exercise. But these daily decisions make all the difference.

You must adopt a mindset that you are going to do what you *need* to do instead of just what you want to do. Only when you place importance on yourself and your health will you begin taking the necessary action steps. No one else can take these steps for you. Not your spouse, not your family, not your doctor — only you!

Mentorship and Accountability

In all areas of life, you excel and succeed when you are accountable and open to guidance and direction. The same is true for your health. Find a mentor, a coach, or a companion in pursuit of your goals.

Popular New Year's resolutions are health-related, whether it's about less eating or more exercising. Frequently, those New Year's resolutions are abandoned two to three weeks into the new year, certainly by Valentine's Day. It's not that these people do not have the desire to get better, or even a small plan of action. They did not have the accountability or the mentorship to guide them through what inevitably happens, which is life and business.

Successful athletes and business executives hire coaches because it allows them to take their game or their business to the next level. These athletes have inherent skills and talents, but sometimes it takes a coach to guide them with their skills or show them how to improve in areas that are being ignored. Like any other goal in life, getting your health where it needs to be often requires an accountability partner, coach, or mentor.

Celebrate Your Victories

If you're like most people, you set ambitious goals — whether it's to lose fifty pounds, or exercise six days a week, or take an inch off your waistline. You put your nose to the grindstone to do what it takes to achieve them. It's not an overnight, quick fix. It requires consistency and patience and the day-in-day-out decision-making.

You may abandon your cause before you've reached your goal, because it seems so far away. The way to succeed is to create smaller, more manageable goals. As you hit these smaller, more manageable goals, you need to celebrate them, embrace them, give yourself that pat on the back, enjoy the process of the journey and achieving these goals.

It's easy to get burned out on the journey if you do not take enough time to celebrate the victories as you accumulate them. If you are looking at health as a journey, which it is, you are going to need to periodically and systematically enjoy these victories.

If you are striving to lose fifty pounds, instead of waiting until your fifty pounds to celebrate, why don't you celebrate at five pounds, ten pounds, fifteen pounds?

Celebration does not have to be food or anything expensive. It can be, and that is fantastic. But just the acknowledgment and enjoyment of the small moment of victory will keep your momentum going and remind you that you are on the right track.

TAKE ACTION

Talk is cheap. You've heard the old saying, *knowledge is powerful*.

I say that knowledge is absolutely worthless unless you are willing to take action with it. Only with action does your knowledge make a difference in your life. You can gather information, scour the Internet, watch videos, and do whatever it takes to gain information, yet you could sit on that information without implementing any of it. You must take action steps to make that knowledge valuable to you.

Define Your Health Goals

Goal setting has been written about, talked about, and embraced by leaders for many decades as being helpful in furthering your endeavors. Setting health goals is just as important to help you achieve what you desire in life. If you don't have a defined goal, then you don't know how to structure your daily activities to achieve what you desire.

Be specific and clear. Put your goal on a timetable.

If your goal is to lose fifty pounds in a year, how many pounds is that per month?

About five pounds. Then you can go smaller and find it's about one pound a week. Now every day, you can make decisions to achieve that one pound a week. A specific and clear plan will dictate all your decisions moment to moment.

If wanted to sail from San Francisco to Hawaii, you'd need to set the coordinates for how to get there. Without charting a course, your chance of getting there is zero. It's only with set coordinates or set goals can you ever expect to achieve the outcome that you seek.

List Three Action Steps to Move Toward Your Goals

Once you have your goal in place, then take action.

If you can define three of the more important steps, that is a good beginning strategy. The process could be brainstorming initially. Write down all the possible action steps you can think of to lead you from where you are to where you want to be. Maybe it's to cut out sugar, or go to bed earlier, or start exercising a couple times a week, or rest and relaxation, or meditation, whatever those action steps could possibly be. Think of as many ideas as you can.

Then go back through the list and find the three that in your opinion will move the needle the absolute most. Start with the thing that will have the most impact. If you can get the ball rolling, especially with the three changes that will have the most impact in your health, then you can gain momentum and add the fourth and the fifth and the sixth. Start with three. Don't start with twenty changes overnight. It will make it much more manageable. When you start getting momentum, it will get easier to add those steps as you move down the path.

Consult Experts

Achieving any major goal in gaining health can be a long, arduous process. Despite your ability to read online or your willingness to do what it takes to get healthy, your willingness to implement plans and get accountability partners, still all of that alone may not bring you completely to the health status or the goal that you truly desire. That is because there is a lot of information and there are a lot of steps. Consulting health experts or well-trained doctors to help you achieve your goal can exponentially speed your process.

When I consult with patients, I remind them that I did not learn by reading a single article or scouring the Internet for a couple of days. I learned through a decade of trial and error, patient interactions, classroom study, and case studies. Now I can help them achieve in six months what took *me* ten years because of the knowledge I gained while becoming an expert.

Despite your best efforts or your own personal motivations, you may be in a situation where you want to take that expert advice. Time is money. If you can achieve your health goals and health status in the fraction of the time than what it would have taken, then you owe it to yourself to do that.

Achieving optimal health is something everyone would like to do. Having an idea to achieve health is only a piece of the puzzle. Not until you are willing to do the action steps can you ever achieve that. I want to encourage you to implement action one step at a time so you can reap the benefits of the knowledge that you gain.

Conclusion

In the grand scheme of things, there is no greater asset an individual can have than their health. Health dictates the ability to enjoy all other blessings that you have in your life. No matter how much money you have, how much free time you have, how many family members, how many loved ones — if you don't have your health, you can't fully enjoy them.

I once heard an old story about a queen who was on her deathbed. She told her physician that she would give him her entire kingdom if he could give her five more minutes of life. This is a great reminder that despite all her wealth and influence and power, at the end of her life, she was willing to abandon all of it for an additional five minutes.

In our fast-paced lives, we don't always remember this truth. We are so caught up with the day-to-day life of family, jobs, responsibilities, and finances that we try to achieve these other things at our own health's expense.

You may think: *I will rest when I'm dead,* or *I will worry about that later.*

You may persistently strive to achieve these things and put your health on a back burner. When you do finally achieve your goals, however, it's not fulfilling because you don't look good, you don't feel good, and you don't enjoy the fruits of your labor to the degree that you could and should because you spent your health.

Not until you prioritize your health will those other things fall into place. When you look at top performers, top athletes, top businessmen, top moms, top dads, everyone will agree that those of us who put health first will find achieving all these other things much easier to do.

As a parent, you may bend over backward trying to achieve things or care for your children at your own expense. It's clearly indicated, however, that if you take care of yourself first, you will be a much better spouse, business owner, father, or mother.

A classic example is turbulence in an airplane and oxygen masks. You are instructed to put the mask on yourself first, and then others. You are much more effective when you care for yourself. Prioritizing health is absolutely necessary.

If you haven't been doing that and have developed a huge health debt, then it is time to start working on paying that off and achieve the health you desire. Just like debt in finances or relationships, it is going to require work, attention to detail, perseverance, and a plan of action to get there.

If you are coming out of a half-million-dollar debt without a plan to repay your debt, it will become difficult to do. The same is true of your health. If you have negated your health for the last ten, fifteen, or twenty years, it will require a plan of action to put the pieces together. It is your responsibility to do so.

You cannot rely on your doctors or the government or your insurance companies to show you what to do; you need to be your own health advocate, reaching out to people you trust and experts to give you guidance. Realize it is going to be a process, not an overnight, quick fix. That is where the tools of setting goals and creating a plan of action are going to be necessary. Identify what your goals are. If they are not defined, crystal clear, and structured with a time frame, it's less likely that you'll take the steps to achieve it.

Imagine in the next three to five years, if you could draw up your perfect health scenario, what would that look like?

How would you feel?

What would your energy levels look like?

How would you sleep?

How would your relationships be?

How would your finances be?

How would your overall life be if your health were exactly where you want it to be in the next three to five years?

Write it in detail. Use that as a vision and as a goal to try to achieve. Basically, once you establish where you want to be, then reverse-engineer it — what will it take to make it happen?

Are there sleep patterns to be improved upon?

Try to create daily steps to move you in that direction. You won't lose all the weight overnight. You won't begin sleeping all night long in the first attempt. Try to find what those goals are and try to find some best practices. Then start achieving them and notice how it feels when you do.

Start small. Start with three or two or even one action step that will move you in that direction. Concentrate on that first.

For example:

- If you drink four sodas a day, knock it down to three.

- If it's exercise, start with walking twenty minutes a day, one day, two days, or three days a week.

- If it's sleep concerns, set a bedtime. If you can't go to sleep before eleven, bump it down to ten. Practice sleep strategies.

There are a lot of resources out there to help you with that. Being conscientious and intentional about achieving your health is what will take you to your next level.

Now that you have all this knowledge, you must apply it through action. Knowledge is worthless unless action is taken. Be willing to start taking those action steps. As you act, remember to give yourself rewards and celebrate the victories. Enjoy the journey.

Often we set out these big, arduous goals and try to achieve them, yet feel empty inside once we achieve them. We realize too late that it's the journey that's fun. Enjoying the days, making this more of a lifestyle, and making conscious decisions every day will help you meet those goals, and more important, keep them.

Embrace that you have the power to dictate your own health. Remember that 95 percent of your current health status has more to do with your health choices than your genetics. You can absolutely achieve the health goals of your dreams!

Next Steps

Talk is cheap!

I hope that the message in this book has served you. My desire is that it educates, empowers, and inspires you to TAKE ACTION! Without action, nothing will change. You owe it to yourself and your loved ones to experience life and health at its fullest potential.

To those of you who are ready to take action and have a desire to jump into the journey of health, then I would like to partner with you and offer guidance.

For some of you, it may be in a capacity of a one-on-one relationship. If this is the case, then I encourage you to contact our office at (704) 588-1792 or visit our website at www.HuntForWellness.com. Due to the wonder of technology we have the privilege of working with individuals all over the globe, and we would love to work with you.

For others, you may simply enjoy some guidance from afar. We encourage you to check out our website at www.HuntForWellness.com and sign up for our newsletter or one of the many FREE reports we have available to you.

For the latest Health News be sure to Like our Facebook page at www.Facebook.com/HuntForWellness.

Thank you for the opportunity to serve you on your Hunt For Wellness!

About the Author

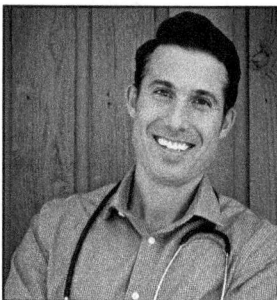

Dr. Tunis Hunt is on a mission to educate, inspire, and empower the world to reach its health potential. A practitioner of health and nutrition since 2005, Dr. Hunt has facilitated change in thousands of lives while building one of the largest wellness clinics in the United States.

The author of three books on health and wellness, Dr. Hunt has helped create guides to a healthier and more balanced life. *The Adrenal Code* focuses on improving vitality, energy, and wellness through understanding the adrenal system and the role it plays in overall health. *The Healthy Detox Diet* creates a guideline for flushing the body of unwanted contaminants. Together, these books aim to educate, inspire, and empower readers to take control of their health.

In addition to working with professional athletes, such as members of the Carolina Panthers, Dr. Hunt has helped countless private patients find the health and wellness they never thought they could have. His process consists of guiding others to uncover their underlying health concerns and create a strategy for regaining the lifestyle they want to have.

Always learning through continued education, journals, and world travel, Dr. Hunt makes the greatest effort to understand the latest research, the most popular trends and their efficacy, and the bio-nutritional guidelines for creating perfect health. He earned his Doctorate in Chiropractic Medicine from Logan University and has dedicated his post-graduate work to fields of Functional Endocrinology, Functional Neurology, Functional Immunology, and Functional Blood Chemistry.

Dr. Hunt has been engaged by some of the largest corporations in the world to share his knowledge on health and wellness. He has given lectures on the subject for corporations such as Sprint, Time Warner, and Belk.

Dr. Hunt is married to Dr. Estela Hunt. Together with their two children, they live a life of practicing what they preach. They keep their health and wellness as their uppermost priority with exercise, a healthy diet, and regular wellness screenings. The Drs. Hunt live and practice in Charlotte, North Carolina.

www.ingramcontent.com/pod-product-compliance
Lightning Source LLC
Chambersburg PA
CBHW052043270326
41931CB00012B/2611